Meniere's Disease

AF485552

OrangeBooks Publication

Smriti Nagar, Bhilai, Chhattisgarh - 490020

Website: **www.orangebooks.in**

First Edition, 2021

ISBN: 978-93-92878-99-2

The opinions/ contents expressed in this book are solely of the author and do not represent the opinions/ standings/ thoughts of OrangeBooks.

Printed in India

MENIERE'S DISEASE

What you need to know

Dr.Anchal Gupta(MBBS, MS ENT)
Dr.Padam Singh Jamwal(MBBS,DLO,MS ENT)

OrangeBooks Publication
www.orangebooks.in

Index

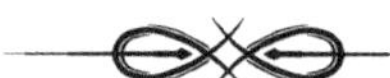

Definition

Meniere's disease is defined as a disease of the membranous inner ear characterised by:

1. Deafness
2. Vertigo
3. Tinnitus

which has as its pathologic correlate hydropic distension of endolymphatic system.

A 4TH symptom AURAL FULLNESS is also added.

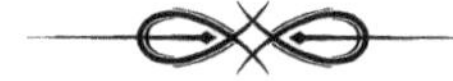

History

150 years & still elusive.....

- In 1747-A ntonio Scarpa described the anatomy of memranous labyrinth

- Prosper Meniere first described the symptom complex in 1861 and proposed the pathologic site to be in the labyrinth.

- In 1871 Knappin advanced the hypothesis that hydrops was similar to ocular glaucoma : aural glaucoma – Knappin theorized that dilated membranous labyrinth to be the cause of this disorder.

- 1927 – Guild described endolymphatic ciruclation

- In 1938 Hallpike and Cairns described the underlying pathology endolymphatic hydrops but the precise etiology still remains elusive

Where do we stand?

1. 150 years have passed since this syndrome was described

2. Amount of literature accumulated has virtually doubled

3. Only consensus reached so far is that its cause is multifactorial

4. *Not all individuals with histological features of Meniere's disease manifested the classic clinical features (? Unknown factors protecting the individuals)*

5. Surgical destruction of sac ameliorates symptoms. *(? What role does sac play exactly in endolymphatic circulation)*

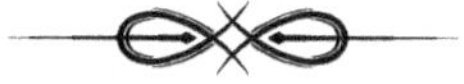

Review Of Anatomy And Physiology

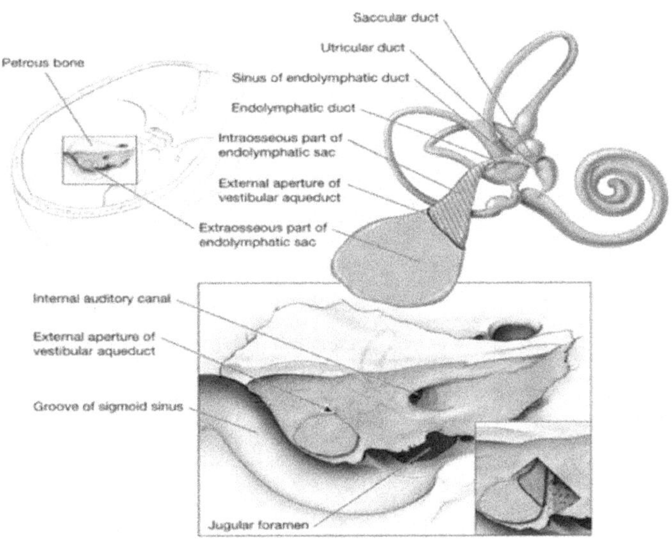

Physiology of inner ear fluids

1. Inner ear contains two types of fluids (perilyimph and endolymph separated by membranous labyrinth.

2. Perilymph is similar in composition to CSF (Containing high Na and low K ions)

3. Endolymph similar in composition to intracellular fluid (Containing low Na and high K concentration). It is secreted by stria vascularis;the planum

semilunatum and dark vestibular cells contribute a small role.

Functions of endolymphatic sac

1. Resorption of the water content of endolymph

2. Ability to participate in some ionic exchanges with endolymph

3. Removal of metabolic and cellular debris, including otoconia

4. Immunodefence function (perisaccular)

5. Inactivation and removal of viruses

6. Secretion of Glycoproteins to attract extra fluid (Glycoproteins act as a driving force for longitudinal flow)

7. Secretion of Saccin to increase Endolymph production

Secretions from the sac

1. Aquaporins

2. Glycoproteins like Saccain

3. Endolymph

4. Glycoproteins act as a driving force for longitudinal flow

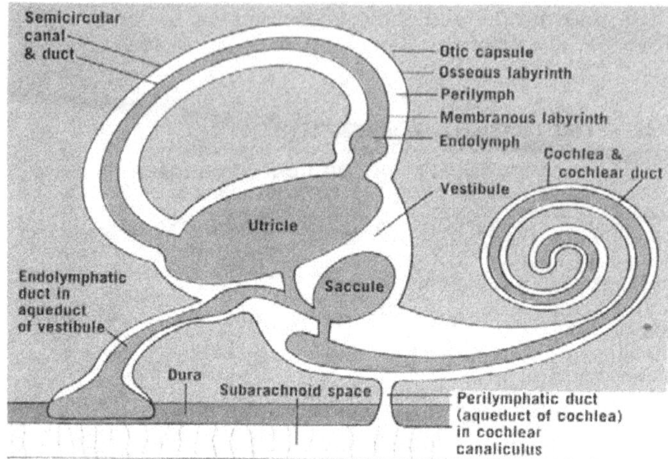

Endolymphatic fluid circulation

1. Longitudinal flow

2. Radial flow

3. Dynamic flow

Longitudinal flow

1. Was first proposed by Guild

2. Striavascularis of cochlea is the principal source.

3. This is a slow process

4. Elimination occurs at the endolymphatic sac level

Dynamic flow

1. First proposed by Lawrence

2. This is a combination of both longitudinal and radial flow patterns

Radial flow

1. This is active process (energy consuming)

2. Production occurs from dark vestibular cells & planum semilunatum

3. Absorption occurs at the striavestibularis

Mechanisms for histopathological changes in menieres disease:

- Fibrosis of endolymphatic sac and vestibular epithelia.

- Altered glycoprotein metabolism.

Inner ear viral infection

Ruptures in menieres disease:

- Endolymphatic hydrops alone is probably not the whole explanation for menieres disease & its related symptoms.

- Ruptures occuring in hydropic membranous labyrinth may be pathophysiological factor.

- The presence of ruptures has led to theory that menieres attacks are due to sudden mixing of endolymph and perilymph and disruption of normal electrochemical activity of the end organ.

- Sensory organs and first order neurons of auditory and vestibular systems are located in perilymph compartment.

- Potassium conc. in endolymph is high about 140mmol/l,a level toxic to neural conductivity.

- A rupture in membranous labyrinth would allow leakage of this neurotoxic endolymph to perilymph resultin in sustained depolarisation and inactivation of hair cells and neurons of 8th nerve. Subsequent healing of membrane rupture and return of endolymph/perilymph barrier would result in return of normal inner ear function and resolution of symptoms of menieres attack.

- Chronic repeated exposure of delicate neural elements of inner ear to endolymph contamination would result in progressive deterioration in auditory and vestibular functions.

- A belief held by some is that high endolymphatic pressure alone can produce menieres symptoms.

Endolymphatic sinus

1. This is a small membranous bulb located where the endolymphatic duct enters the vestibule

2. This is where the volume of circulating endolymph is monitored

3. Monitoring the volume of endolymph is not possible by sac because it will be interfered by CSF pressure and pressure exerted by lateral sinus

How endolymphatic sinus monitors endolymph volume

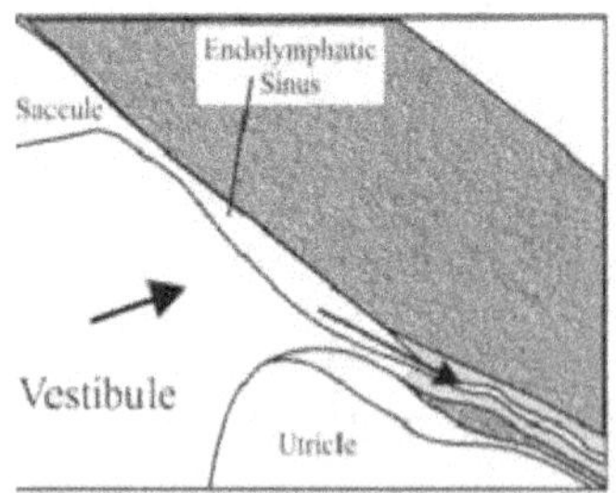

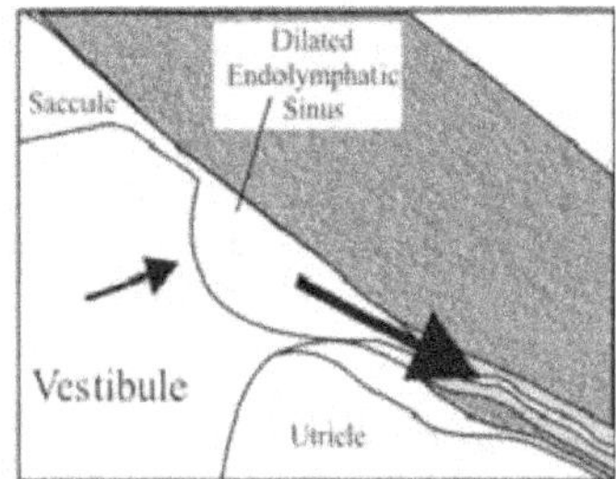

Schematic of how the endolymphatic sinus detects and regulates endolymph volume status. When endolymph volume is normal (left), pressure elevations in the vestibule (black arrow) produce only small endolymph movements into the sac before the sinus membrane occludes the duct. In contrast, when the endolymphatic sinus is dilated (right), pressure elevations in the vestibule result in a larger volume being forced into the sac before the duct is occluded. The increase in volume delivered to the sac with dilation of the endolymphatic sinus will act to counteract the volume increase, acting to stabilize endolymph volume within a specific range.

Salt's findings on endolymphatic flow

1. Composition of endolymph is maintained by stria vascularis by controlling the influx of water

2. Normally endolymph is a biological puddle with very little radial / longitudinal flow

3. Only under exceptional circumstances like increased endolymphatic fluid volumes does radial / longitudinal movement towards sac occurs

4. Under normal circumstances radial flow alone is sufficient to maintain endolymph fluid balance and the longitudinal flow due to saccmechanics is not necessary

5. The longitudinal flow is restricted by the isthmus portion of the duct which acts like the constriction seen in the hour glass

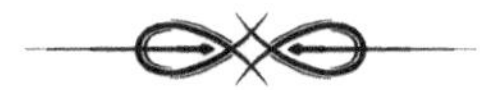

Aetiopathology

Idiopathic

B. Increased production of endolymph:

- Allergy

- Sodium & water retention

- Autoimmune

- Viral infection

- sympathetic activity → ischemia of stria

  vascularis → fluid transudation

Endocrine → Hypo (thyroidism, pituitarism,

adrenalism), Diabetes, Hyperlipoproteinemia

C. Decreased absorption of endolymph:

- Small size of endolymphatic sac / duct

- Obstruction of endolymphatic sac / duct

- Ischaemia of endolymphatic sac

- Inner ear trauma

- Genetic- AD

- Immunological - immune complex deposition

- Viral-serum IgE to herpes simples virus types I and II, Epstein-Barr virus and CMV

- Vascular-associated with migraines

- Metabolic-potassium intoxication

- Meniere's Disease is associated with several abnormalities of the temporal bone, including hypoplasia of the vestibular aqueduct. The endolymphatic sac is small and can lie in an abnormal position below the labyrinth. A pedigree study by Morrison yielded a

- family history in 7.7% with an autosomal dominant mode of inheritance for Meniere's Disease.

- The endolymphatic sac is osmotically and immunologically active. Evidence of immune complex deposition In the endolymphatic sac in patients with Meneire's disease

- Has reinforced the belief that the disease is an immune disorder.

- The role of neurotropic viruses is conflicting. Calenoff et al showed specific IgE

- To herpes simplex types I and II and Epstein-Barr virus and cytomegalovirus in the serum of patients with Meniere's disease.

- Metabolic causes include potassium intoxication. The endolymph is a potassium rich hyperosmolar fluid that is positively charged with respect to perilymph. Maintenance of his ionic milieu depends on the activity of sodium potassium ATPase in the stria vascularis of the cochlear duct. In Meniere's disease there is distention if the endolymphatic sac leading to potassium intoxication which leads to chronic loss of hair cell motility and deafness.

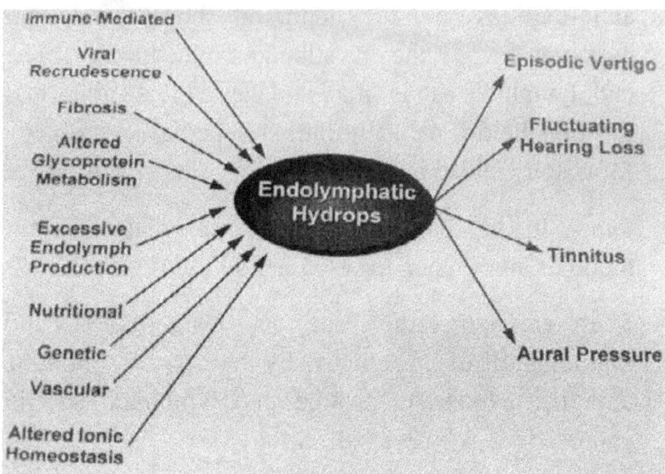

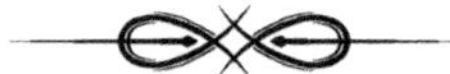

Pathophysiology

- Menieres disease appears to be one member of a group of disorders of the inner ear linked by common pathophysiological condition of endolymphatic hydrops.

- Endolymphatic hydrops is thought to be a pathological condition that is the end result of a variety of insults to the inner ear,and may be subdivided into :

- Symptomatic

- Asymptomatic forms.

Classification of endolymphatic hydrops

Symptomatic	Asymptomatic
Embryopathic	Embryopathic
Acquired • postinflammatory • post traumatic	Acquired • postinflammatory • post traumatic
Idiopathic	Idiopathic

- The symptomatic form is characterised by classical triad of fluctuating hearing loss, episodic vertigo and usually tinnitus and the asymptomatic form is clinically silent.

- **Endolymphatic hydrops is physical distortion in membranous labyrinth.**

- **Cochlear hydrops**-seen in all cases

- **Saccular hydrops-**most cases

- **Utricular hydrops-**uncommon.

- Endolymphatic hydrops was therefore seen most consistently in pars inferior & could be identified by typical boeing of Reissners membrane and distension of saccule.

- Enlargement of endolymphatic space occurred at the expense of perilymphatic space.

- Fibrous adhesions form between saccule and stapedial footplate.

- This contact may explain **Hennebert's Sign** (subjective vertigo nystagmus observed during pressure induced excursion of footplate.

- It may also explain **Tullio Phenomenon** (subjective imbalance and nystagmus observed in response to loud,low frequency noise exposure.)

- Despite the progressive decline in auditory and vestibular functions observed in these patients over years, there is relative sparing of first order neurons and only in most severe cases will these structures show damage and depletion in numbers.

Drainage theory
1. Small amounts of excess endolymph can be cleared by radial flow

2. Larger volumes need longitudinal flow for their clearance

3. Endolymphatic sinus temporarily accommodates excess endolymph till the sac is ready for it

4. Endolymphatic valve of Bast isolates pars superior and prevents endolymph from draining out of the utricle

5. Endolymphatic hydrops leads to rupture of membranous labyrinth as a result of which potassium rich endolymph mixes with perilymph . This causes sustained inactivation of hair cells & neurons of vestibulo-cochlear nerve bathed in perilymph leading to deafness + vertigo + tinnitus

6. Increased Sympathetic activity causes ischemia of cochlear & vestibular end organs hence leading to deafness + vertigo.

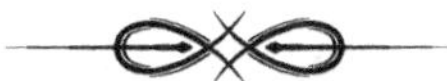

Epidemiology

Incidence and prevalence

The exact incidence and prevalence of Ménière's disease are unknown and in fact difficult to demonstrate in any population because of inherent difficulties to diagnose this condition after exclusion of all other possible causes.

First-line physicians tend to overdiagnose Ménière's disease in patients with chronic vertigo (with or with- out recurrent vertigo or any additional symptoms). In a secondary or tertiary referral balance clinic it is difficult to establish the exact catchment area.

The age of onset is more commonly reported in the second to sixth decade of life. Only 1–7% of Ménière's disease cases are seen in the paediatric population.

Surprisingly, 9% of all patients experience the start of Ménière's disease at the age of 65 or more, with a higher incidence of drop

Sex

There is no difference in the female-to-male ratio.

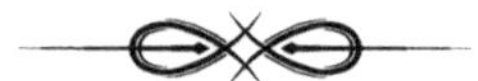

Clinical Manifestations

---

1. Episodic vertigo rotatory in nature
2. Ipsilateral hearing loss
3. Aural fullness
4. Roaring tinnitus
5. Diplacusis

Episodic Vertigo

- The attacks of vertigo may be preceded by an aura consisting of aural fullness,increasing tinnitus and hearing loss lasting 15-60 mins.

- The length of attack is variable with most episodes lasting 2-3 hrs.

- The clinical rule of thumb that attacks of vertigo in menieres disease last **'24 Minutes To 24 Hours'** is valid for majority of cases.

- Episodic vertigo associated with vegetative signs like nausea vomitting is most stressing and disabling symptom.

- Vertigo begins suddenly with severe spinning sensation & is accompanied by pallor, diaphoresis, nausea, diarrhea & vommiting.

- During the attack patient has a normal level of consciousness and orientation and suffers no focal neurological symptom.

- Over the following minutes to hours symptoms gradually subside & patient often falls asleep.

- Following the attack patients often feel normal.

- Some may complain of dysequilibrium, light headedness or motion intolerance most commonly in first 24 hrs.

Lermoyez syndrome

This is a variant of Meniere's disease. The vertiginous episode is preceded by increasing tinnitus and hearing loss but unlike the classic condition hearing loss or tinnitus dramatically resolve during or shortly after the onset of dizziness.

An explanation to its pathophysiology is lacking.

Tumarkin's drop attacks

This variant is characterized by abrupt falling attacks of brief duration without loss of consciousness.

Patient describe a sensation of being pushed or thrown to ground or a sudden illusion of movement of environment. This is caused due to an enlarging utricle due to excess endolymphatic volume. Utricular crisis is used to indicate this condition.

In the later disease stages the valve of Bast remaining patent may cause sudden drainage of endolymph from the utricle due to longitudinal flow resulting in these drop attacks

Abnormal oculovestibular response

- Another variant of menieres disease.

- These patients experience vertigo with its vegetative symptoms of nausea,vomitting and diaphoresis when exposed to optokinetic stimuli such as riding in a car or train.

- Most of them also had other symtoms of menieres disease.

Menieres disease and BPPV

- 85.9% of patients complain of positional vertigo between attacks of menieres disease.

- Unlike the definitive spells of vertigo these attacks are short lived lasting seconds only and are provoked by certain head movements.

- Patient may present with classical history of menieres disease and have classical BPPV finding of rotatory nystagmus on Dix-hallpike testing.

Aetiology of BPPV in menieres disease:

- Free floating particles in posterior scc and repostioning of these particles into utricle resluts in resolution of vertigo.

- In menieres disease these particles may be generated by coalescence and concretion of endolymhatic glycoproteins or inflammatory products seen in temporal bone studies or there may be otoconia dislodged by metabolic or degenerative changes occuring in sensory organs of vestibule.

NYSTAGMUS IN menieres:

- Acute attacks are rarely observed by physician but if they are HORIZONTAL NYSTAGMUS is classical physical finding.

- **Irritative Nystagmus:** A near instantaneous recording in the caloric test position captures a nystagmus beating towards the affected ear for 20 seconds.

- **Paralytic Nystagmus:** nystagmus then beats towards the healthy ear after very short time.

- **Recovery Nystagmus:** nystagmus reverses again beating towards the affected side after hours into attack when auditory and vestibular symptoms subside.It may be horizontal or rotatory.

Sensorineural Hearing Loss

- Fluctuant and progressive.

- Hearing may fluctuate significantly in first year or two.

- During acute spell auditory acuity is always decreased and remains so for sometime after vertigo has subsided.

- Early in the disease characteristic pattern is of low frequency fluctuant hearing loss.

- Second early pattern is of low frequency hearing loss occuring in concert with high frequency hearing loss resulting in inverted V pattern on audiogram at 2KHZ

- HEARING LOSS TENDS TO FLATTEN WITH TIME.

- The average pure tone hearing loss over long term is 50db with speech discrimination score of 53%.

- The decrease in hearing acuity is typical of cochlear type of sensorineural hearing loss.

- DIPLACUSIS BINAURALIS DYSHARMONICA; the same sound frequency is perceived as a different pitch in the two ears with the affected ear perceiving a higher pitch.

- Loudness intolerance due to recruitment is another common feature.

- RECRUITMENT: oversensitivity to suprathreshold acoustic stimulus is a manifestation of hair cell injury and is absent in the lesions of auditory nerve.

Tinnitus

- Variable in character.

- May be the first symptom of disorder and it may begin with attack.

- Always present during the spell.

- May be continuous or intermittent .

- Non pulsatile.

- Pitch corresponds to region of most severe hearing loss and severity is loosely related to severity of hearing loss.

- Earlier in the disease it becomes loud and then softer as hearing improves.

- Later it may be constant and more distracting between attacks.

Variants Of Meniere's Disease

1. Classical Meniere's disease

2. Vestibular Meniere's disease – vestibular symptoms and aural pressure

3. Cochlear Meniere's disease – cochlear symptoms and aural pressure

4. Lermoyez syndrome – Reverse Meniere's

5. Tumarkin's crisis – Utricular Meniere's

Central	Peripheral	Metabolic
• Acoustic neuroma • Multiple sclerosis • Vascular loop compression syndrome • Aneurysm	• BPPV • Labyrynthitis • Perilymphatic fistula • Otosclerosis • Migraine induced vertigo	• Diabetes • Hyper/hypo thyroidism • Syphilis • Cogan's syndrome • Anemia • Autoimmune disorders

<ul><li>Vascular insufficiency</li><li>Arnold-chiari malformation</li><li>Cerebellar or brainstem tumors</li><li>Cervical vertigo</li><li>Transient ischemic attacks/ CVA</li></ul>	23	

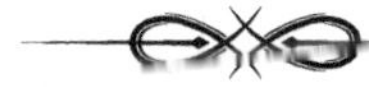

Differential Diagnosis

Stahle and Klockhoff divided differential diagnosis of menieres into :

✓ Conditions with vertigo without auditory symptoms

✓ Conditions with auditory symptoms without vertigo

✓ Conditions with a combination of auditory symptoms and vertigo

Conditions With Vertigo Without Auditory Symptoms

- Vestibular neuronitis

- Benign Paroxysmal Positional Vertigo (BPPV)

Vestibular Neuronitis

- Characterised by change in the vestibular output of one inner ear,resulting in severe vertigo.

- The patient is very ill initially and vertigo and vegetative symptoms subside over 24-48 hrs ,time taken for central compensation to occur.

- Mild attacks of vertigo may persist for 2months and sometimes upto 6 months.

- Patients are more prone to travel sickness and motion intolerance.

- The length of attack and lack of auditory symptoms or aural fullness distinguish it from menieres disease.

BPPV

- Evoked by changes in head position.

- An attack is usually triggered when patient lies back on affected side,rolls over onto that side,sits up quickly or tilts the head back while looking up.

- A latent period of some sec. after head movement is followed by severe vertigo which usually lasts less than 1 min

- Dix-hallpike testing is positive when a rotatory nystagmus is induced with the affected ear dependant,a response which is fatiguable.

Conditions With Auditory Symptoms Without Vertigo

- Sudden deafness

- Vestibular schwannomas/acoustic neuroma

Sudden Deafness

- Sudden deafness is distinguished from initial stages of menieres disease by the fact that hearing loss develops more quickly usually across a frequency spectrum.

- Aural fullness is usually absent.

Vestibular Schwannomas

Usually presents with progressive sensorineural hearing loss and often tinnitus.

Rotatory vertigo is unusual and patients complain of dysequilibrium.

PTA shows high frequency hearing loss.

The absence of recruitment,very poor dicrimination and absent stapedial reflex or marked stapedial reflex decay may be present and differentiates from menieres disease.

2% of patients present with classical menieres triad of symptoms including rotatory vertigo.

- Secondary endolymphatic hydrops can occur in patients with vestibular schwannomas perhaps relating to high CSF protein.

All patientsshould have the diagnosisof a vestibular schwannomas excluded by MRI with gadolinium DTPA enhancement

Diagnosis

Physical Examination

- Examination results vary, depending upon the phase of disease.

- During an acute attack, the patient has severe vertigo.

- Spontaneous nystagmus directed toward affected ear is typical during an acute attack.

    1. Irritative nystagmus during the first 20 mins of attack

    2. Paralytic nystagmus follows

Later recovery nystagmus starts

- The Romberg test generally shows significant instability and worsening when the eyes are closed.

- The Weber tuning fork test usually lateralizes away from the affected ear.

- The Rinne test usually indicates that air conduction remains better than bone conduction.

- Complete neurologic evaluation is important. New-onset vertigo might be an early sign of stroke, migraine, or brainstem compression that may require emergent evaluation and care.

Routine Tests

- Audiometry (with speech discrimination test and impedance testing)

- Electronystagmography with caloric testing

- Auditory brainstem response

- Radiographs of the mastoid

- Laboratory tests (hemogram, erythrocyte sedimentation rate,thyroid, cholesterol, triglycerides, glucose,fluorescent treponemal antibody absorption test)

Extended tests

- Electrocochleography (ECOG)

- Glycerol test (with audiometry with tests of distortion product otoacoustic emissions or ECOG)

- Vestibular autorotation test

- Video-oculography

- Traveling-wave velocity technique

- Autoimmune tests

- Glucose tolerance test with measurement of insulin in plasma

- Computed tomography scan

- Magnetic resonance imaging

Pure Tone Audiometry
Particularly helpful to document present hearing acuity and to detect future change.

-The patient may not notice a loss at specific frequencies. Low-frequency or mixed low- and high-frequency insufficiency may be observed.

- Typically, the lower frequencies are affected more severely. This is due to preferential sensitivity of the apex to the hydrops.

- Multiple hearing tests, which document fluctuating hearing loss, are helpful in diagnos. The audiometric presentation of a patient with Meniere's disease can be variable. Most of the time it can be seen as a sensorineural hearing loss with several different configurations and, occasionally, as a conductive loss (at very early stages of the disease when there is still good cochlear performance) or a mixture of both (mixed loss) during bouts of hydrops ing Ménière.

This conductive component maybe the reason why so many patients with Meniere's disease who suffer a feeling of aural fullness and have an air-bone gap shown on audiometry have been mistakenly treated with insertion of ventilation tubes.

The early stages of the disease tend to be associated with low-frequency sensorineural hearing loss. At later stages, very often the hearing loss progresses to a flat pattern. Very frequently, the authors have seen loudness recruitment and reduced speech discrimination.

A pattern of low-frequency fluctuating loss and a coincident nonchanging, high-frequency loss is described, resulting in a "peaked" or "tent-like" tracing on the audiogram. This peak classically occurs at 2 kHz.

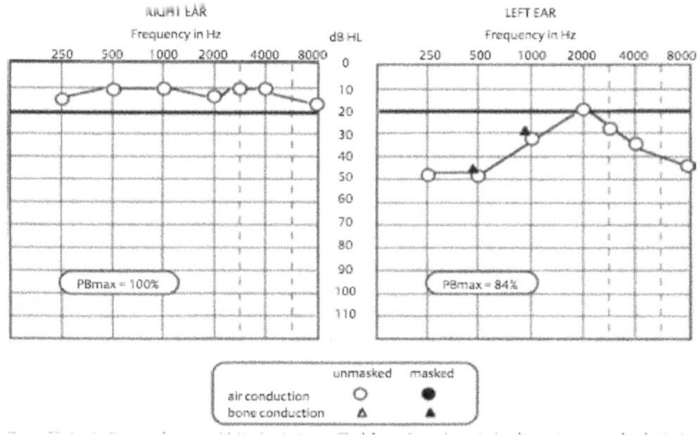

Audiogram typical of early Meniere's disease on the right side (x=left, o=right). There is a low-tone sensorineural hearing loss

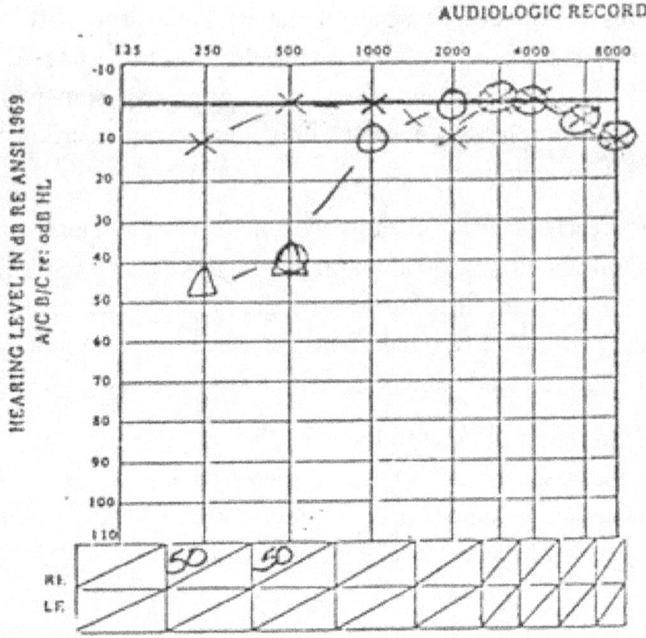

Imaging Studies

- Magnetic resonance imaging

- R/o abnormal anatomy or mass lesions. Specifically, acoustic neuromas or CP angle lesions. Other lesions, such as multiple sclerosis or Arnold-Chiari malformations, also can be ruled out.

- CT scans reveal dehiscent superior semicircular canals and/or widened cochlear and vestibular aqueducts

Other SPECIAL INVESTIGATIONS

- Electronystagmography

- Head Thrust Testing

- Electrocochleography

- Dehydrating Agents

- Vestibular evoked Myopotentials

Electronystagmography

- Electrooculographic recordings of eye movements after caloric and rotational stimulation are a commonly available and reliable method of assessing vestibular function.

- The caloric test often can localize the involved ear. A significant caloric response reduction is found in 48% to 73.5% of patients with Meniere's disease.

- As many as 25% of meniere's disease patients have no abnormalities

- *Electronystagmography with caloric testing*

- Vestibular testing should include at least spontaneous, gaze, saccade, smooth pursuit, rotatory, and caloric testing. Even though spells of vertigo constitute the most disruptive symptom of Meniere's disease, vestibular examination will often demonstrate a normal result in these patients. Results of routine vestibular testing are highly nonspecific for Meniere's disease and may fluctuate with time for any patient. Spontaneous and positional nystagmus is frequently seen and has no value in predicting which ear is hydropic.

There are two possible explanations for the low sensitivity of vestibular testing in Meniere's disease. The initial stage of the disease could represent a low functional impairment of the vestibular organ and, beyond that, there is the fact that vestibular tests only partially evaluate vestibular function because only the horizontal vestibular semicircular canal is assessed. The most important finding, however, from any vestibular test in Meniere's disease is still unilateral vestibular hypofunction, measured by caloric testing , even though up to 50% of patients with Meniere's disease will have normal findings, even in the presence of incapacitating vestibular symptoms.

Radiographs of the mastoid

- Routine mastoid radiographs (Schuller's view) to

- Verify the presence of changes in pneumatization of the mastoid process.

- It is important to know whether the mastoid is sclerotic, diploic, or pneumatic.. Some authors have described mastoid and periaqueductal

- hypocellularity in Meniere's disease .

Head Thrust Testing

- The head thrust test popularized by Halmagyi is very sensitive for detection of unilateral vestibular dysfunction.

- However, in Meniere's disease, the asymmetry is subtle and present in only 29% of the patients.

Vestibular Evoked Myopotentials

- VEMPs are generated by playing loud clicks in the ear, which move the stapes footplate and stimulate the saccule. This is the start of a disynaptic pathway that passes through the vestibular nuclei and then to synapses that relax the sternocleomastoid muscle.

- The saccule is the second most common site affected by hydrops, which has caused VEMPs to be investigated as a potential diagnostic tool. In the normal ear, the best response is near 500 Hz.

- Ears affected by Meniere's disease have elevated VEMP thresholds with flattened tuning.

- The interaural amplitude difference in the response has been implicated as a staging tool for Meniere's disease.

- Although these tests show differences between populations, they currently have limited diagnostic value owing to the large individual variation in responses.

- Other Audiological Tests

- Speech Audiometry: Score = 50 - 80 %

- Alternate binaural loudness balance test (ABLB): Recruitment present

- Short increment sensitivity index (SISI): positive (> 70 % score)

- Tone Decay Test: negative (decay < 20 dB)

Transtympanic Electrocochleography:

- Most satisfactory potentials in terms of amplitude are obtained from middle ear promontory near the round window niche or via a silver ball electrode placed on the round window.

- This method involves placement of a thin ,teflon coated 0.3mm dia stainless steel needle electrode through the tympanic membrane,which has been anaesthetised using iontophores.

- Sound stimuli are produced from a loudspeaker in earphones.

- *The Cochlear Microphonic Potential* sound energy is transduced in the inner ear from mechanical vibration of basilar membrane into electrical energy by hair cells.

- *The Summating Potential* is a potential of short latency and is usually only present at high stimulus intensities. The summating potential is a complex multicomponent response representing sum of various electrical events occuring within the cochlea.

Electro-cochleography findings in Meniere's disease

- Summation potential : compound action potential ratio > 30 %

- Widened SP-AP waveform (> 2msec)

- Small Distorted cochlear micro-phonics

- Widening of SP/AP is a very useful measure of degree of endolymphatic hydrops.

Applications of electrocochleography:

- Continuous transtympanic electrocochleographic recording during glycerol dehydration in patients with menieres disease demonstrates a significant decrease in width of SP.

- It may confirm the diagnosis of menieres disease when it is in prevertiginous stage.

- Useful in identifying incepient disease in the second ear in patients with documented unilateral disease.

- In syphilis AP/SP complex is W-shaped with an enhanced negative summating potential notch. Preop electrocochleography is of value in selecting patients for surgery and is of prognostic value.

- Monitoring electrophysiological changes occuring in cochlea and 8th nerve in menieres disease in response to therapeutic modalities and surgery.

- Intraoperatively used to monitor the progress of endolymphatic sac surgery.

SP – AP Waveform

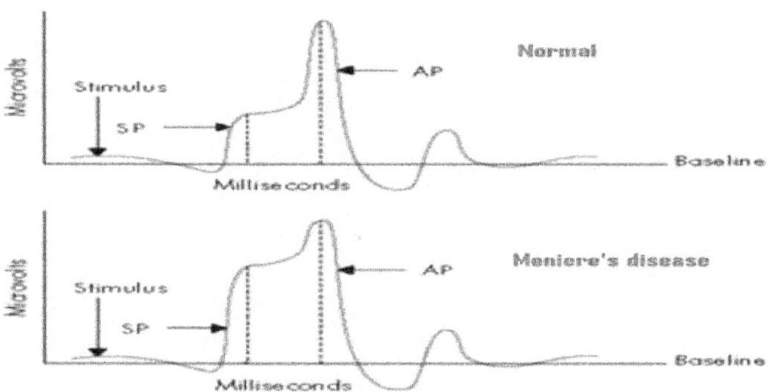

Cochlear Microphonics

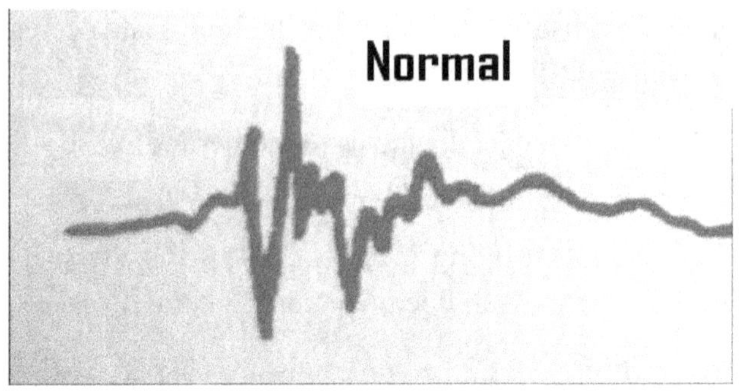

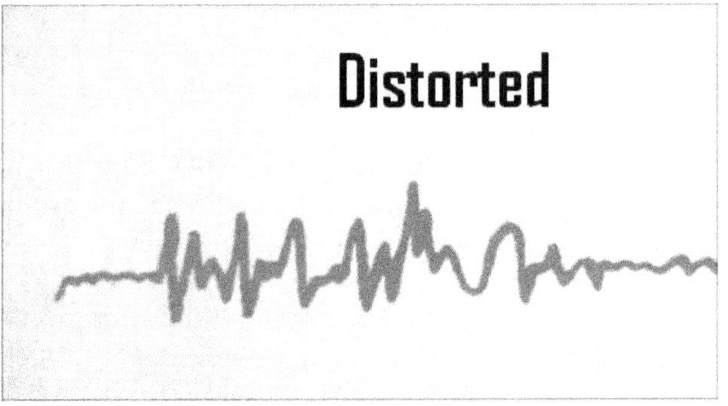

Glycerol Test (confirmatory)

- Do P.T.A. & speech audiogram. Glycerol (1.5 ml / Kg), mixed in lime juice given orally. Repeat audio tests after 2 hrs. Test is positive if:

- Pure Tone threshold improves > 10 dB

- Speech Discrimination Score increases > 15 %

- S.P. / A.P. ratio in E.Co.G. decreases > 15 %

Reverse Glycerol Test

- ACETAZOLAMIDE, a carbonic anhydrase inhibitor has been used to increase the cochlear endolymphatic hydrops.

- Documentation of deterioration in pure tone thresholds and speech discrimination scores and increase in the enhancement of negative summating action potential following acetazolamide supports diagnosis of menieres disease.

Other Investigations

- Full blood count + ESR

- Urea, electrolytes

- RBS, FBS

- Fasting lipid profile

- Thyroid function test

- VDRL, TPHA

- Immunological assay, antibody screening

AAO-HNS Criteria for Meniere's Disease Diagnosis
Major Symptoms

1. Vertigo
   - Recurrent, well-defined episodes of spinning or rotation • Duration from 20 minutes to 24 hours.
   - Nystagmus associated with attacks
   - Nausea and vomiting during vertigo spells common
   - No neurologic symptoms with vertigo

2. Deafness
   - Hearing deficits fluctuate

- Sensorineural hearing loss

- Hearing loss progressive, usually unilateral

3. Tinnitus

   - Variable, often low-pitched and louder during attacks

   - Usually unilateral

   - Subjective

4. Possible Meniere's disease

   - Episodic vertigo without hearing loss or

   - Sensorineural hearing loss, fluctuating or fixed, with dysequilibrium, but without definite episodes

   - Other causes excluded

   - Probable Meniere's disease

   - One definitive episode of vertigo

   - Hearing loss documented by audiogram at least once

   - Tinnitus or sense of aural fullness in the presumed affected ear

   - Other causes excluded

   - Definite Meniere's disease

   - Two or more definitive spontaneous episodes of vertigo lasting at least 20 minutes

   - Audiometrically documented hearing loss on at least one occasion

- Tinnitus or sense of aural fullness in the presumed affected ear

- Other causes excluded

- Certain Meniere's disease

- Definite Meniere's disease, plus histopathologic confirmation

AAO-HNS Criteria for Meniere's Disease Severity
Vertigo

a) Any treatment should be evaluated after at least 24 months.

b) Formula to obtain numeric value for vertigo:

ratio of average number of definitive spells per month after therapy divided by definitive spells per month before therapy (averaged over a 24-month period) $\times$ 100 = numeric value.

Numeric value scale	Control	Class
0	Complete control of definitive spells	A
0-40	Limited control of definitive spells	B
41-80	Insignificant control of definitive spells	C
81-120		D
>120	Secondary treatment initiated	E

Disability

a) No disability

b) Mild disability: intermittent or continuous dizziness/unsteadiness that precludes working in a hazardous environment.

c) Moderate disability: intermittent or continuous dizziness that results in a sedentary occupation

d) Severe disability: symptoms so severe as to exclude gainful employment

Hearing

1. Hearing is measured using a four-frequency pure-tone average (PTA) of 500 Hz, 1 kHz, 2 kHz, and 3 kHz.

   - Pretreatment hearing level: worst hearing level during 6 months before therapy

   - Post-treatment hearing level: poorest hearing level measured 18-24 months after institution of therapy

2. Hearing classification:

   - Unchanged: ≤10-dB PTA improvement or worsening or ≤15% speech discrimination improvement or worsening.

   - Improved: >10-dB PTA improvement or >15% discrimination improvement

   - Worse: >10-dB PTA worsening or >15% discrimination worsening

3. In 1996, the Committee on Hearing and Equilibrium reaffirmed and clarified the guidelines, adding initial staging and reporting guidelines:

4.   Initial Hearing Level

Stage	Four tone average
1	≤ 25
2	26-40
3	41-70
4	>70

Functional Level Scale

Regarding my current state of overall function, not just during attacks:

- My dizziness has no effect on my activities at all.

- When I am dizzy, I have to stop for a while, but it soon passes and I can resume my activities. I continue to work, drive, and engage in any activity I choose without restriction. I have not changed any plans or activities to accommodate my dizziness.

- When I am dizzy I have to stop what I am doing for a while, but it does pass and I can resume activities. I continue to work, drive, and engage in most activities I choose, but I have had to change some plans and make some allowance for my dizziness.

- I am able to work, drive, travel, and take care of a family or engage in most activities, but I must exert a great deal of effort to do so. I must constantly make adjustments in my activities and budget my energies. I am barely making it.

- I am unable to work, drive, or take care of a family. I am unable to do most of the active things that I used to do. Even essential activities must be limited. I am disabled.

- I have been disabled for 1 year or longer and/or I receive compensation because of my dizziness or balance problem.

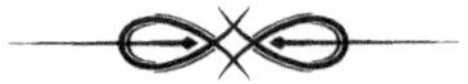

Treatment

Total labyrinthectomy
Vestibular neurectomy
Ultrasonic vestibular destruction
Chemical labyrinthectomy
Endolymphatic sac surgery
Meniett device
Cinnarizine
Betahistine
Salt restriction
Destructive
Conservative
Diagnosis confirmed
All patients
Low salt diet, avoidance of caffeine, chocolate, alcohol, tobacco products
3-6 month trial
Acute attack
Diuretics
Oral, intramuscular, or intratympanic steroids
Treatment failure
Meniett device
Treatment failure
Endolymphatic sac enhancement surgery
Treatment failure
Gentamicin perfusion
Treatment failure
Vesticular neurectomy
Treatment failure
Labyrinthectomy

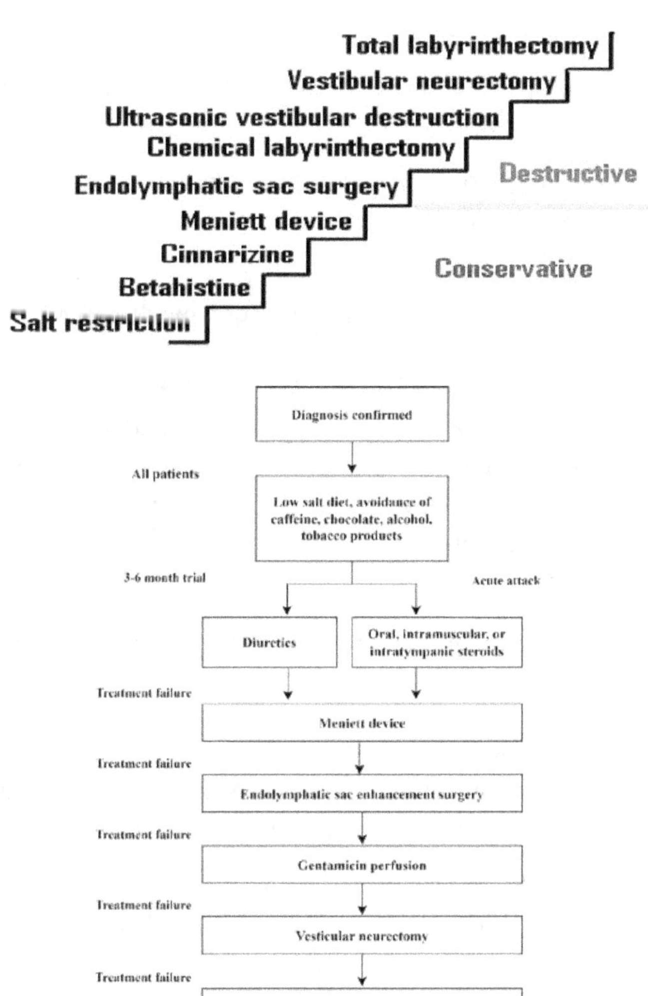

Medical Management

1. Dietary management
2. Physiotherapy
3. Psychological support
4. Pharmacological intervention

Medical Treatment

- A good doctor patient relationship is of paramount importance.

- Patient is very apprehensive and requires considerable support and reassurance.

Psychological support is possibly the most important aspect of medical treatment of this chronic disorder

Symptomatic Relief During Acute Episodes:

- **Vestibular Suppressants:** acute vertigo during an attack of menieres disease is due to sudden asymmetry in vestibular input to CNS. These drugs are well established in controlling vertigo and vegetative symptoms.

- They have variable anticholinergic, antiemetic and sedative properties.

These include

- **Phenothiazines:** prochlorperazine(inj.stemetil 12.5mg i.v. t.id or q.i.d) and perphenazine

- **Antihistaminics:** cinnarizine, cyclizine, dimenhydrinate, promethazine hydrochloride (phenergan 25mg i.v. t.i.d or q.i.d) and meclizine hydrochloride.

- **Benzodiazepines:** lorazepam and diazepam(calmpose 5mg i.v. stat).

- **Others Are:** transdermal scopolamine hydrobromide (an anti-Ach that crosses BBB) and ASTEMIZOLE(doesnot cross BBB)

Prophylaxis Between Acute Episodes

- Discussion: Reassurance. Avoid tea, coffee, colas, chocolate, allergens, stress, smoking, alcohol, flying, diving, heights.

- Diet: Low salt (1.5 g/day), less fluids.

- Exercise.

- Vestibular Depressants: Cinnarizine, Diazepam, Prochlorperazine, Dimenhydrinate.

- Cochlear VasoDilators: Betahistine, Xanthinol nicotinate, Carbogen (5 % CO2 + 95 % O2), L.M.W. Dextran, Histamine drip.

- Diuretics: Thiazide + Triamterene

- Dexamethasone / Ig G: decreases auto-immunity

- Dehydration by hyperosmolar fluids

- Hormone replacement therapy.

- Carbonic anhydrase inhibitors e.g.acetazolamide were initially recommended because of presence of carbonic anhydrase in endolymph producing dark cells and stria vascularis(s/e:increases hydrops and hearing loss)

Role of diuretics

1. Diuretics play a vital role in alleviating acute symptoms

2. This has been in use since 1930's

3. Thiazide group of drugs are commonly used

4. Frusemide may be used to alleviate acute symptoms

5. Clear scientific evidence is lacking regarding the usefulness of diuretics (cochrane review)

Betahistine

1. Cochlear vascular insufficiency has been proposed as one of the mechanism of Meniere's disease

2. Betahistine is supposed to cause vasodilatation of cochlear blood vessels

3. Betahistine has weak H1 agonistic property and considerable H3 antagonist properties

4. It reduces the frequency & intensity of vertigo. Has minimal effect on tinnitus

5. Doesn't help much with hearing loss (Cochrane review)

6. Other vasodilators include: papaverine, isoxsuprine,nylidrin, dipyridamole, amyl nitrite, nitroglycerine, nicotinic acid, co2 & thymoxamine

Intratympanic steroids

1. Immune modulating effects

2. Improves fluid dynamics of inner ear due to mineralocorticoid effects

3. Vertigo was controlled on an immediate basis

4. Methylprednisolone has the best effect as it penetrates the round window better

Silverstein microwick can be used for intratympanic drug administration

Other treatments:
- Steroids

- Cytotoxic drugs

- Lymphocytoplasmaphoresis

- immunoglobulinG

- Methyl B12

- Acupuncture and herbal preparations

- Hypobaric pressure chamber therapy

- Hearing loss is generally rehabilitated through the use of hearing aids.

- Tinnitus is treated with reassurance and masking

- Tinnitus clinics and self help groups can be very helpful.

- Vestibular rehabilitation is also recommended in some cases.

Vibrator therapy
1. Meniett Device

2. Low pressure pulse generator

3. Vibrations are transmitted via external auditory canal

4. Vibrations alter inner ear fluid dynamics by their effects on the oval and round windows

5. Exact mechanism of action is not known

6. It is totally non invasive

7. This device is portable.

Vibrator therapy steps

1. Diagnosis should be confirmed

2. Ventilation tube should be inserted

3. Patient should be trained for self administration of the treatment

4. Usually administered thrice a day about 5 mins each time

5. Treatment lasts for 5 weeks

Indications for vibrator therapy

1. Classic unilateral Meniere's disease

2. Intense vestibular / cochlear symptoms

3. Failed medical therapy

4. Over 65 years of age

5. Imbalance / aural fullness / tinnitus after gentamycin treatment

Surgical Treatment Of Meniere's Disease

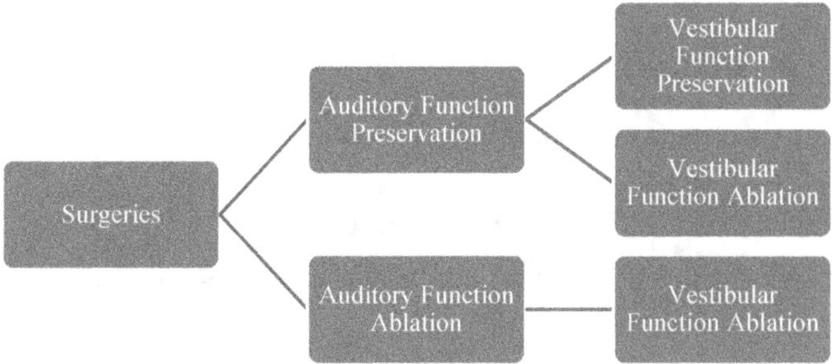

A. Hearing preservation + Balance preservation:
1. Endolymphatic sac decompression / shunting

2. Sacculotomy by puncture of footplate

3. Cochlear duct piercing via round window

B. Hearing preservation + Balance ablation:
1. Chemical labyrinthectomy

2. Vestibular neurectomy

3. Vestibular end organ destruction by USG / cryoprobe

C. Hearing ablation + Balance ablation:
1. Section of 8th nerve

2. Total labyrinthectomy

Decompression Surgery
1. Endolymphatic sac decompression (Portmann)

2. Endolymphatic sac shunting: into subarachnoid space or mastoid cavity

3. Sacculotomy:

- Fick's needle puncture of footplate

- Cody's tack puncture of footplate

4. Cochlear duct piercing via round window

Fick And Cody Tack Procedures

- Were designed to create fistula in the saccule via oval window.

- The Fick procedure accomplished this through direct manipulation of saccule with a pick via the oval window.

- Cody procedure involved insertion of a sharp 1.5mm tack through the membranous attachments of stapes footplate.

- Now abandoned because of inconsistent results and their high incidence of hearing loss.

Endolymphatic sac decompression

Endolymphatic sac surgery begins with simple mastoidectomy and identification of the tegmen, sigmoid sinus, and facial ridge. Once these landmarks are established, the horizon¬tal and posterior canals should be skeletonized and the bone over the posterior fossa thinned. Only a thin covering of bone should be left over the facial nerve and the sigmoid sinus to allow adequate exposure of the posterior fossa dura. The bone over the posterior fossa should be completely removed using a diamond bur .The endolymphatic sac lies on the dura medial to the vertical segment of the facial nerve and the retrofacial air cells. The superior aspect of the endolymphatic sac should be identified, and often lies just below a line (Donaldson's line) formed by extending the plane of the horizontal semicircular canal posteriorly to bisect the posterior semicircular canal. The procedure from this point varies according to which endolymphatic surgery is planned. Decompression of the sac requires only that the bone of the pos¬terior fossa plate be removed.

Endolymphatic shunting is most simply performed by incis¬ing the exposed sac and placing a stent to keep the incision open. The popular Paparella and Hanson technique involves open¬

ing the edge of the sac, lysing any intraluminal adhesions, and probing the duct to insure that it is patent. A piece of "Silastic" is placed through the incision i n the sac allowing long-term drain¬age .

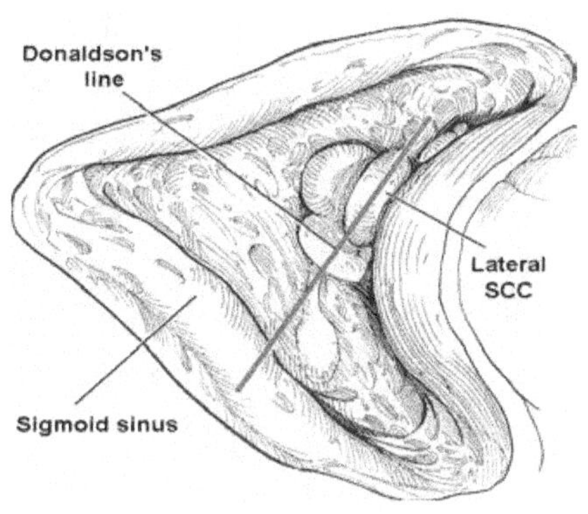

Endolymphatic sac decompression

Sac shunting into mastoid and subarachnoid spaces

Shunting the sac into the subarachnoid space is more elab¬orate since it requires making a second incision in the poste¬rior wall of the endolymphatic sac into the posterior fossa and a specially designed shunt tube.After the initial, lateral incision is made in the sac, a small medial incision is made to allow a shunt to be placed into the basal cistern creating a passage into the subarachnoid space. The resulting CSF leak is controlled by placing a fascia graft over the lateral incision in the sac. Obliteration of the mastoid cavity with an abdominal fat graft is also an option. This technique has not been as popular in recent years due to its relative complexity, the higher risk of a postoperative CSF leak, and intracranial hematoma as a result of drainage to arachnoid veins.

All of these procedures can be performed in an outpatient center, and patients can usually return to work within a week,¬ a recovery rate similar to mastoidectomy alone. Although the procedure is intended to be a hearing-sparing procedure with minimal morbidity, the risk of hearing loss may be as high as 5%. In addition, there is a small risk of facial nerve damage associated with the procedure.

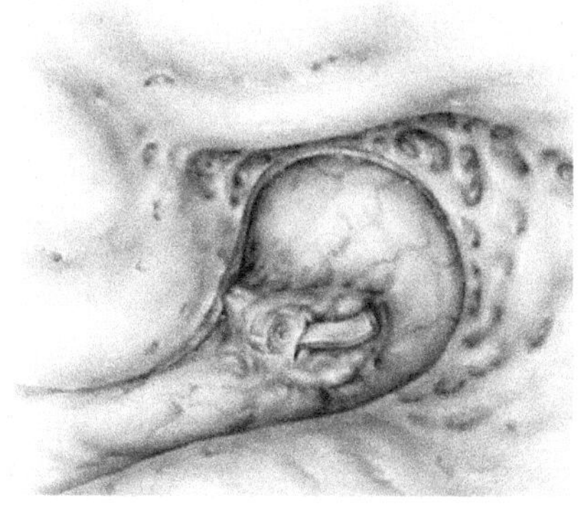

Sac shunting into mastoid

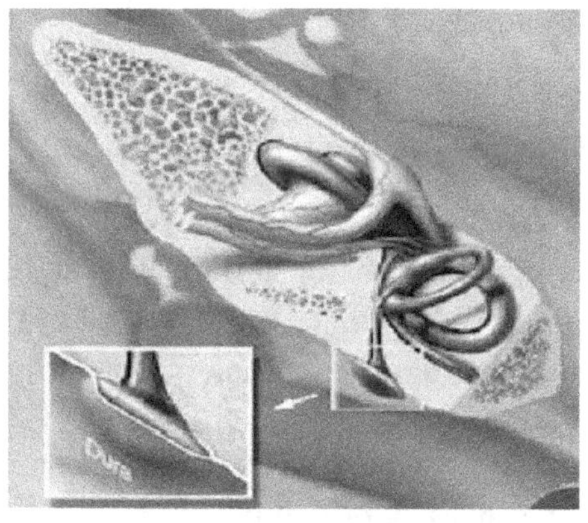

Sac shunting into subarachnoid

Tenotomy of the tensor tympani and stpedial muscle tendons

Conflicting results have been reported on tenotomy of the tensor tympani and stapedial muscles' tendons. The suggested mechanism of action in Ménière's disease patients is that the tympanic membrane is pushed laterally by increased cochlear pressure against the ossicular chain.

By sectioning the tensor tympani muscle this effect is (partially) alleviated.

Procedures Involving Ablation Of 8th Nerve:

- Via suboccipital approach

- Exposure of internal auditory meatus through the middle cranial fossa:advantage of this procedure is ease with which vestibular nerve can be differentiated from the cochlear and facial nerves in lateral internal auditory meatus allowing greater accuracy of nerve section and decreasing the likelihoodof injury to hearing and facial movement.

- Transtemporal supralabrynthine approach.

- Retrosigmoid approach: involves sectioning of superior vestibular and posterior ampullary nerves via the retrosigmoid approach after removal of some bone from the posterior aspect of internal auditory meatus.

Chemical Labyrinthectomy
Trans-tympanic drug injection

- Intra-tympanic drug instillation via grommet

- Intra-tympanic drug instillation via Silverstein micro wick

- Trans-tympanic drug perfusion

Drug used: Gentamicin (vestibulotoxic)

Trans-tympanic gentamicin
- 26.4mg/ml solution used

- 0.8 ml solution instilled in affected ear (via T-tube iserted into tympanic membrane and attached to tubal apparatus or grommet) 3 times daily for 4 consecutive days for a total of 12 doses or 208mg.

- After instillation, pt to lie supine with affected ear up for 30 min & not swallow anything

- Vertigo control = 94%. Hearing unchanged or improved = 74%. Hearing worsened = 26%.

Indication

- Active unilateral menieres disease with frequent disabling attacks of vertigo which have not responded to conservative medical management.

  contraindications:

- Pre existing tympanic membrane perforation.

- Active inflammation of middle ear.

- Allergy to aminoglycosides.

- Impaired renal function.

- High risk of poor post-procedural central nervous system compensation.

- Menieres disease in an only hearing ear.

  Perilymphatic space application of aminoglycoside:

  Involves perfusion of inner ear with 100microgram of streptomycin via an opening created in the horizontal semicircular canal,followed by intramuscular injection of 1 microgram of streptomycin.

Parenteral aminoglycosides:

- Used in bilateral menieres disease.

- Objective of this treatment is reduction or elimination of vertigo with maximal hearing preservation.

- Titrated doses of parenteral streptomycin in amounts upto 20 grams and with monitoring of vestibular function during therapy.

Trans-tympanic Dexamethasone
Mechanism of action:

- reducing inflammation

- control of auto-immune injury

   Solution strength: 0.25 mg/ml

   Dose: 5 drops every alternate day for 3 months

   Total Destructive Surgery

   Destroys both cochlear & vestibular functions.

   Done in pt with severe deafness.

   Types of surgery are:

- Section of vestibular + cochlear nerves

Total labyrinthectomy- Labyrinthectomy is the Most destructive procedure in the treatment of Meniere's as it destroys both hearing and vestib¬ular function. Ideal candidates for labyrinthectomy are those who have no hearing and have failed more conservative treat¬ tnents, such as gentamicin injection. Despite its morbidity, the procedure has a higher rate of vertigo control than vestibular neurectomy. There are two approaches: transcanal and transmastoid, although the transmastoid approach affords much better exposure and is more popular.

How Can I Prevent Meniere's Disease?
No measures will prevent Meniere's disease, but you can take preventive measures to avoid or minimize attacks and consequences of attacks.

- Reduce salt in your diet.

- Stop smoking.

- Avoid Alcohol and Caffeine

- Avoid exposure to loud noises.

- Manage stress.

- Use caution at home and on the job to avoid falling or having an accident if you feel dizzy.

Dietary and lifestyle changes in Meniere's Disease

The following dietary and lifestyle changes may lessen the severity and frequency of Meniere's disease symptoms.

Limit salt intake. Foods and beverages high in salt can increase fluid retention. Persons with Meniere's disease should aim for $1,500 mg of sodium each day.

Avoid monosodium glutamate (MSG). MSG, which contains sodium, can contribute to fluid retention. Some packaged food products and prepared restaurant foods contain MSG.

Avoid caffeinated foods and beverages. Chocolate, coffee, tea, and certain soft drinks have stimulant properties that can make symptoms worse. For instance, caffeine may make tinnitus louder.

Eat regular meals. Even distribution of food and drink throughout the day helps regulate body fluids. Eat approximately the same amount of food at each meal.

Quit smoking. Avoiding nicotine may reduce the severity of Meniere's disease symptoms.

Manage stress and anxiety. It is not known whether stress and anxiety act as triggers for Meniere's disease symptoms or are the result of having the disorder. Professional counseling may help patients identify stressors and develop strategies for coping with stress and anxiety. Medications to alleviate anxiety may also be beneficial.

Avoid allergens. There are reports of an association between allergies and Meniere's disease. Controlling exposure to allergens and seeking appropriate treatment to manage allergies may also help manage Meniere's disease.

Prevent migraine. Evidence is emerging that links Meniere's disease and migraine, suggesting that migraine management may lessen the severity of Meniere's disease.

References

1. Committee on Hearing and Equilibrium guidelines for the diagnosis and evalu- ation of therapy in Meniere's disease. Otolaryngol Head Neck Surg 1995; 113(3): 181–5.

2. Kotimäki J, Sorri M, Aantaa E, Nuutinen J. Prevalence of Meniere disease in Finland. Laryngoscope 1999; 109(5): 748–53.

3. Ballester M, Liard P, Vibert D, Hausler R. Meniere's disease in the elderly. Otol Neurotol 2002; 23(1): 73–8.

4. 4. Fransen E, Verstreken M, Verhagen WI, et al. High prevalence of symptoms of Meniere's disease in three families with a mutation in the COCH gene. Hum Mol Gen 1999; 8(8): 1425–9.

5. Verstreken M, Declau F, Wuyts FL, et al. Hereditary otovestibular dysfunction and Meniere's disease in a large Belgian family is caused by a missense mutation in the COCH gene. Otol Neurotol 2001; 22(6): 874–81.

6. Kawaguchi S, Hagiwara A, Suzuki M. Polymorphic analysis of the heat-shock protein 70 gene (HSPA1A) in Meniere's disease. Acta Otolaryngol 2008; 128(11): 1173–7.

7. Foster CA, Breeze RE. Endolymphatic hydrops in Meniere's disease: cause, conse- quence, or epiphenomenon? Otol Neurotol 828 Section 2: The Ear

8. Yamane H, Takayama M, Sunami K, et al. Blockage of reuniting duct in Meniere's disease. Acta Otolaryngol 2010; 130(2): 233–9.

9. Merchant SN, Adams JC, Nadol JB Jr. Pathophysiology of Meniere's syndrome: are symptoms caused by endolymphatic hydrops? Otol Neurotol 2005 Jan; 26(1): 74–81.

10. Bernstein JM, Shanahan TC, Schaffer FM. Further observations on the role of the MHC genes and certain hearing disorders. Acta Otolaryngol 1996; 116(5): 666–71.

11. Gacek RR. Meniere's disease is a viral neu- ropathy. ORL J Otorhinolaryngol Relat Spec 2009; 71(2): 78–86.

12. Derebery MJ. Allergic management of Meniere's disease: an outcome study. Otolaryngol Head Neck Surg 2000; 122(2): 174–82.

13. Kimura R. Experimental endolymphatic hydrops. In: Harris JP (ed.). Meniere's disease. The Hague: Kugler Publications; 1999, pp. 115–24.

14. Lopez-Escamez JA, Carey J, Chung WH, et al. Diagnostic criteria for Meniere's disease. J Vestibular Res 2015; 25(1): 1–7.

15. Bance M, Mai M, Tomlinson D, Rutka J. The changing direction of nystagmus in acute Meniere's

disease: pathophysiological implications. Laryngoscope 1991; 101(2): 197–201.

16. Schuknecht HF, Gulya AJ. Endolymphatic hydrops: an overview and classification. Ann Otol Rhinol Laryngol Suppl 1983; 106: 1–20.

17. Godemann F, Siefert K, Hantschke- Bruggemann M, et al. What accounts for vertigo one year after neuritis vestibu- laris – anxiety or a dysfunctional vestibular organ? J Psychiatr Res 2005; 39(5): 529–34.

18. Neff BA, Staab JP, Eggers SD, et al. Auditory and vestibular symptoms and chronic subjective dizziness in patients with Meniere's disease, vestibular migraine, and Meniere's disease with concomitant vestibular migraine. Otol Neurotol 2012; 33(7): 1235–44.

19. Lempert T, Olesen J, Furman J, et al. Vestibular migraine: diagnostic criteria. J Vestibular Res 2012; 22(4): 167–72.

20. Hufner K, Barresi D, Glaser M, et al. Vestibular paroxysmia: diagnostic features and medical treatment. Neurology 2008; 71(13): 1006–14.

21. Staab JP, Ruckenstein MJ, Amsterdam JD. A prospective trial of sertraline for chronic subjective dizziness. Laryngoscope 2004; 114(9): 1637–41.

22. Wuyts FL, Van de Heyning PH,Van Spaendonck MP, Molenberghs G. A review of electrocochleography: instru- mentation settings and meta-analysis of criteria for diagnosis of

endolymphatic hydrops. Acta Otolaryngol Suppl 1997; 526: 14–20.

23. De Valck CF, Claes GM, Wuyts FL,Van de Heyning PH. Lack of diagnostic value of high-pass noise maskingof auditory brainstem responses in Meniere's disease. Otol Neurotol 2007; 28(5): 700–7.45. Shang YY, Diao WW, Ni DF, et al. Study of cochlear hydrops analysis masking proce- dure in patients with Meniere's disease and otologically normal adults. Chin Med J 2012; 125(24): 4449–53.

24. Hong SK, Nam SW, Lee HJ, et al. Clinical observation on acute low-frequency hearing loss without vertigo: the role of cochlear hydrops analysis masking proce- dure as initial prognostic parameter. Ear Hear 2013; 34(2): 229–35.

25. Liu F, Huang W, Meng X, et al. Comparison of noninvasive evaluation of endolymphatic hydrops in Meniere's dis- ease and endolymphatic space in healthy volunteers using magnetic resonance imaging. Acta Otolaryngol 2012; 132(3): 234–40.

26. Nakashima T, Naganawa S, Pyykko I,et al. Grading of endolymphatic hydrops using magnetic resonance imaging. Acta Otolaryngol Suppl 2009; 560: 5–8.

27. Arroll M, Dancey CP, Attree EA, et al. People with symptoms of Meniere's disease: the relationship between illness intrusiveness, illness uncertainty, dizziness handicap, and depression. Otol Neurotol 2012; 33(5): 816–23.

28. Friscia LA, Morgan MT, Sparto PJ, et al. Responsiveness of self-report measuresin individuals with vertigo, dizziness, and unsteadiness. Otol Neurotol 2014; 35(5): 884–8.

29. Kato BM, LaRouere MJ, Bojrab DI, Michaelides EM. Evaluating qual- ity of life after endolymphatic sacsurgery: the Meniere's Disease Outcomes Questionnaire. Otol Neurotol 2004; 25(3): 339–44.

30. Bodmer D, Morong S, Stewart C, et al. Long-term vertigo control in patients after intratympanic gentamicin instillation for Meniere's disease. Otol Neurotol 2007; 28(8): 1140–4.

31. Dineen R, Doyle J, Bench J, Perry A. The influence of training on tinnitus perception: an evaluation 12 months after tinnitus management training. Br J Audiol 1999; 33(1): 29–51.

32. Claes J, Van de Heyning PH. A review of medical treatment for Meniere's disease. Acta Otolaryngol Suppl 2000; 544: 34–9.

33. James AL, Burton MJ. Betahistine for Meniere's disease or syndrome. Cochrane Database Syst Rev 2001; (1): CD001873.

34. Nauta JJ. Meta-analysis of clinical studies with betahistine in Meniere's disease and vestibular vertigo. Euro Arch Otorhinolaryngol 2014; 271(5): 887–97.

35. Lezius F, Adrion C, Mansmann U, et al. High-dosage betahistine dihydrochloride between 288 and 480 mg/day in patients with severe Meniere's disease: a

case series. Euro Arch Otorhinolaryngol 2011; 268(8): 1237–40.

36. Ingelstedt S, Ivarsson A, Tjernstrom O. Immediate relief of symptoms during acute attacks of Meniere's disease, using a pressure chamber. Acta Otolaryngol 1976; 82(5-6): 368–78.

37. Basile AS, Huang JM, Xie C, et al. N-methyl-D-aspartate antagonists limit aminoglycoside antibiotic-induced hearing loss. Nat Med 1996; 2(12): 1338–43.

38. Wu WJ, Sha SH, Schacht J. Recent advances in understanding aminoglycoside ototoxicity and its prevention. Audiol Neurootol 2002; 7(3): 171–4.

39. Tepel M. N-Acetylcysteine in the preven- tion of ototoxicity. Kidney Int 2007; 72(3): 231–2.

40. Schuknecht HF. Ablation therapy for the relief of Meniere's disease. Laryngoscope 1956; 66(7): 859–70.

41. Schuknecht HF. Ablation therapy in the management of Meniere's disease. Acta Otolaryngol Suppl 1957; 132: 1–42.

42. Pullens B, van Benthem PP. Intratympanic gentamicin for Meniere's disease or syn- drome. Cochrane Database Syst Rev 2011; (3): CD008234.

43. Huon LK, Fang TY, Wang PC. Outcomes of intratympanic gentamicin injection to treat Meniere's disease. Otol Neurotol 2012; 33(5): 706–14.

44. Casani AP, Piaggi P, Cerchiai N, et al. Intratympanic treatment of intractable unilateral Meniere disease: gentamicin or dexamethasone? A randomized controlled trial. Otolaryngol Head Neck Surg 2012; 146(3): 430–7.

45. Viana LM, Bahmad F, Jr., Rauch SD. Intratympanic gentamicin as a treatment for drop attacks in patients with Meniere's disease. Laryngoscope 2014; 124(9): 2151–4.

46. Pullens B, Giard JL, Verschuur HP, van Benthem PP. Surgery for Meniere's disease. Cochrane Database Syst Rev 2010; (1): CD005395.

47. Sood AJ, Lambert PR, Nguyen SA,Meyer TA. Endolymphatic sac surgery for Meniere's disease: a systematic review and meta-analysis. Otol Neurotol 2014 ; 35(6): 1033–45.

48. Silverstein H, Smouha E, Jones R. Natural history vs. surgery for Meniere's disease. Otolaryngol Head Neck Surg 1989; 100(1): 6–16.

49. Loader B, Beicht D, Hamzavi JS, Franz P. Tenotomy of the stapedius and tensor tympani muscles reduces subjective dizziness handicap in definite Meniere's disease. Acta Otolaryngol 2013; 133(4): 368–72.

50. Jang CH, Park H, Choi CH, et al. The effect of increased inner ear pressure on tympanic membrane vibration. Int J Pediatr Otorhinolaryngol 2009; 73(3): 371–5.

51. Hillman TA, Chen DA, Arriaga MA. Vestibular nerve section versus intratympanic gentamicin for

Meniere's disease. Laryngoscope 2004; 114(2): 216–22.

52. Colletti V, Carner M, Colletti L. Auditory results after vestibular nerve section and intratympanic gentamicin for Meniere's dis- ease. Otol Neurotol 2007; 28(2): 145–51.

53. Schmerber S, Dumas G, Morel N, et al. Vestibular neurectomy vs. chemical laby- rinthectomy in the treatment of disabling Meniere's disease: a long-term comparative study. Auris Nasus Larynx 2009; 36(4): 400–5.

54. D'Agostino RB, Sr. The delayed-start study design. N Engl J Med 2009; 361(13): 1304–6.

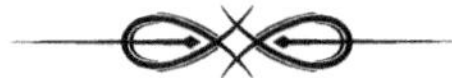